This publication is intended to provide educational information for the reader on the covered subjects. It is not intended to take the place of personalized medical counseling, diagnosis, and treatment from a trained healthcare professional.

ISBN 978-1-998455-97-3 (Paperback)
ISBN 978-1-998455-98-0 (eBook)

Printed and bound in USA
Published by Loons Pre

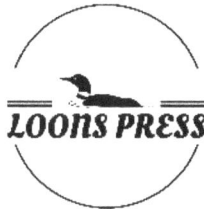

I0106280

LOONS PRESS

Table Of Contents

Chapter 1   **6**

Understanding Floaters   **6**

What Are Floaters?   6

Causes of Floaters   9

Types of Floaters   12

When to Seek Medical Attention   14

Chapter 2   **18**

The Anatomy of the Eye   **18**

Structure of the Eye   18

The Vitreous Humor   21

How Floaters Form in the Eye   23

Chapter 3   **28**

Assessing Your Floaters   **28**

Identifying Symptoms   28

Self-Assessment Techniques   30

Keeping a Floaters Diary   33

Chapter 4   **37**

Lifestyle Changes for Eye Health   **37**

    Nutrition for Eye Health   37

    Hydration and Its Importance   40

    The Role of Exercise   43

Chapter 5   **47**

Natural Remedies for Floaters   **47**

    Herbal Supplements   47

    Essential Oils   50

    Homeopathy   52

Chapter 6   **56**

Eye Exercises   **56**

    Importance of Eye Exercises   56

    Basic Eye Exercises   58

    Advanced Techniques   61

Chapter 7   **65**

Medical Treatments   **65**

    Laser Therapy   65

    Vitrectomy   68

Alternative Medical Approaches | 70

Chapter 8 | **75**

Preventive Strategies | **75**

Regular Eye Check-Ups | 75

Protecting Your Eyes from Harm | 77

Managing Eye Strain | 80

Chapter 9 | **84**

Coping with Floaters | **84**

Emotional and Psychological Impact | 84

Mindfulness and Relaxation Techniques | 87

Building a Support Network | 90

Chapter 10 | **94**

Future Research and Innovations | **94**

Advances in Eye Care Technology | 94

Potential Breakthroughs in Treatment | 97

Staying Informed on Eye Health Trends | 100

Author Notes & Acknowledgments | **104**

Author Bio | **106**

How To Heal Floaters

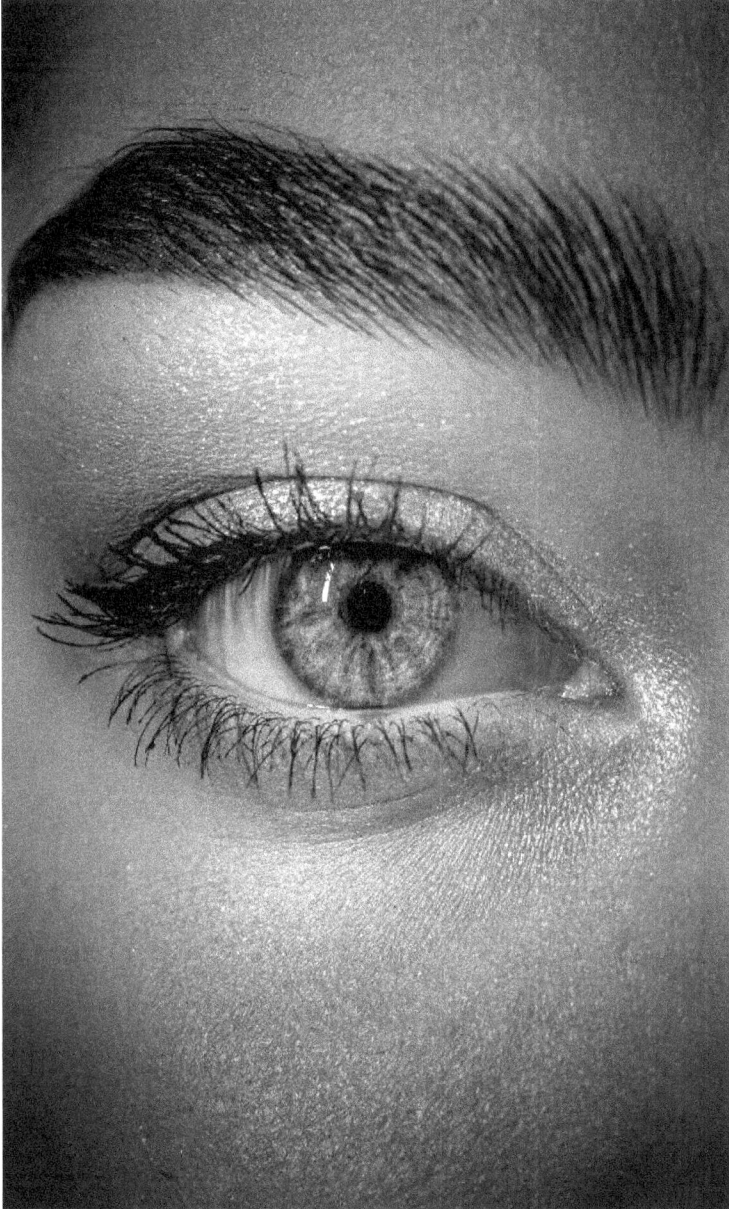

Chapter 1

Understanding Floaters

What Are Floaters?

Floaters are small, shadowy shapes that can appear in a person's field of vision, often resembling cobwebs, specks, or squiggly lines. They are typically more noticeable against bright backgrounds, such as a clear sky or a white wall.

Floaters are caused by tiny clumps of gel or cells inside the vitreous, the gel-like substance that fills the eye. As we age, the vitreous can shrink and become more liquid, leading to the formation of these floaters.

Most floaters are benign and a common part of the aging process, but understanding their nature is essential for determining when they may warrant further investigation.

The appearance of floaters is often a normal phenomenon, especially for individuals over the age of 50. However, newcomers to floaters may find them alarming, particularly if they notice a sudden increase in their number or changes in their visibility. While many people learn to ignore floaters over time, they can sometimes be indicative of underlying issues with the retina or vitreous.

If a person experiences a sudden increase in floaters, especially if accompanied by flashes of light or peripheral vision changes, it is crucial to seek medical attention. Such symptoms could signal a more serious condition, such as a retinal tear or detachment.

Floaters can come in various shapes and sizes, and their movement can be influenced by eye movement. When a person looks around, floaters may drift and shift, often leading to frustration as they seem to follow the gaze. This phenomenon is due to their position in the vitreous; they float in the gel-like substance and are perceived as moving when the eye moves.

Over time, many people adapt to floaters, learning to ignore them as they become a regular part of their visual experience. However, for some individuals, floaters can be distracting or bothersome enough to seek treatment or management strategies.

In terms of treatment, there are limited options available for floaters, primarily because they are often harmless. In some cases, laser therapy may be used to break up larger floaters, making them less noticeable.

However, this approach is not universally recommended since it carries its own risks and may not be effective for everyone. Vitrectomy, a surgical procedure that involves removing the vitreous gel along with its floaters, is another option but is typically reserved for severe cases due to potential complications. For most people, learning to cope with floaters might be the most practical approach.

Preventive measures for floaters focus on overall eye health. Maintaining a healthy lifestyle, which includes a balanced diet rich in antioxidants, regular exercise, and avoiding smoking, can contribute to better eye health and potentially reduce the risk of developing floaters.

Regular eye examinations are also crucial, as they allow for early detection of any changes in eye health. While floaters are often a benign part of aging, staying informed about eye health and changes in vision can empower individuals to take proactive steps and seek appropriate care when necessary.

Causes of Floaters

Floaters are often described as small specks, cobwebs, or thread-like strands that drift across the field of vision. Understanding the causes of floaters can empower individuals to address their concerns and seek appropriate solutions. The primary cause of floaters is age-related changes in the vitreous humor, the gel-like substance that fills the eye.

As we age, the vitreous can become more liquid and may begin to separate from the retina. This separation can lead to the formation of tiny clumps of gel or fibers, which cast shadows on the retina, resulting in the perception of floaters.

Another common cause of floaters is the presence of posterior vitreous detachment (PVD). This condition occurs when the vitreous gel pulls away from the back of the eye. While PVD is often a normal part of aging, it can lead to an increase in floaters as the gel shifts and clumps together.

Individuals experiencing PVD may notice a sudden increase in floaters, accompanied by flashes of light. Although PVD is typically harmless, it is essential to have a thorough eye examination to rule out more serious conditions.

Inflammation within the eye, known as uveitis, can also lead to the development of floaters. Uveitis can occur due to various factors, including autoimmune diseases, infections, or previous eye injuries. In this case, the inflammation can cause debris to form within the vitreous, resulting in floaters that can affect vision. Prompt medical attention is critical for managing uveitis and preventing potential complications.

Additionally, other eye conditions such as retinal tears or detachments can produce floaters. When the retina is damaged or detached, it can lead to the release of cells and fluid into the vitreous cavity, contributing to the appearance of floaters. This situation is considered a medical emergency, as it can lead to vision loss if not treated promptly. Understanding the signs and symptoms of retinal issues can help individuals seek timely intervention.

Lastly, systemic conditions such as diabetes and high blood pressure can impact eye health and contribute to the presence of floaters. Diabetic retinopathy, a complication of diabetes, can lead to changes in the retina and vitreous, resulting in floaters.

Maintaining overall health through proper management of chronic conditions is vital in reducing the risk of floaters and protecting eye health. Being aware of these causes enables individuals to take proactive steps in seeking treatment and improving their eye health.

Types of Floaters

Floaters are tiny spots, lines, or cobweb-like structures that drift across the field of vision, often becoming more prominent in bright light. Understanding the types of floaters can help individuals better recognize their symptoms and seek appropriate strategies for treatment. Floaters are generally classified into two main categories: vitreous floaters and retinal floaters. Each type has its own characteristics and implications for eye health.

Vitreous floaters are the most common type, resulting from changes in the vitreous gel, the clear substance that fills the eye. As people age, the vitreous can become less gel-like and more liquid, leading to clumps or strands that cast shadows on the retina.

These floaters may appear as small dots, squiggly lines, or cobwebs and can vary in size and opacity. While they are typically harmless, an increase in the number or size of these floaters can indicate changes in the vitreous that warrant further examination by an eye care professional.

Retinal floaters, on the other hand, are often associated with more serious conditions. These floaters occur when there is an issue with the retina, such as a tear or detachment. Retinal floaters can manifest suddenly and may be accompanied by flashes of light or a curtain-like shadow in the peripheral vision.

Unlike vitreous floaters, retinal floaters require immediate medical attention, as they may signify a risk of vision loss. Understanding the distinction between these two types is crucial for those concerned about floaters, as it can inform their response and actions.

Another category worth mentioning is inflammatory floaters, which result from inflammation in the eye, often linked to conditions such as uveitis. Inflammatory floaters may appear suddenly and can be accompanied by redness, pain, or sensitivity to light. This type of floater indicates an underlying issue that needs to be addressed, as the inflammation can lead to more severe complications if left untreated. Individuals experiencing these symptoms should seek prompt professional evaluation to determine the cause and appropriate treatment.

Lastly, post-surgical floaters are a consideration for those who have undergone eye surgery, such as cataract removal or vitreous surgery. These floaters can develop as a result of changes in the eye's internal structures following surgical intervention. While many people find that their floaters diminish over time, some may continue to experience them long after recovery.

Understanding the types of floaters and their implications is essential for individuals concerned about their eye health, enabling them to take proactive steps toward managing their symptoms and seeking appropriate care.

When to Seek Medical Attention

Understanding when to seek medical attention for eye floaters is crucial for maintaining optimal eye health. Floaters are often harmless and a common occurrence as we age, but certain signs may indicate a more serious underlying condition. Recognizing these signs early can help prevent potential complications and ensure timely treatment. This subchapter will outline specific scenarios in which seeking professional help is essential.

If you experience a sudden increase in the number of floaters, it is vital to consult an eye care professional immediately. This sudden change can signify a retinal tear or detachment, which requires urgent attention. Retinal detachment can lead to permanent vision loss if not treated promptly.

If you notice a significant change in your floaters, such as their size, shape, or behavior, do not hesitate to schedule an appointment.

Another important sign to watch for is the presence of flashes of light accompanying your floaters. These flashes, often described as stars or lightning streaks, can suggest that the retina is being pulled or stretched.

This phenomenon, known as posterior vitreous detachment, may lead to complications if not monitored by a specialist. If you notice these flashes, especially if they are new or worsening, it is advisable to seek medical evaluation.

In addition to changes in floaters, any sudden loss of vision or blurry vision warrants immediate medical attention. These symptoms can indicate a range of serious conditions, including retinal detachment, vitreous hemorrhage, or other ocular diseases. A thorough examination by an eye care professional can help determine the cause of these symptoms and the appropriate course of action.

Finally, if you have a history of eye disease or conditions such as diabetes or high blood pressure, you should be particularly vigilant. Individuals with these conditions are at a higher risk for developing complications related to floaters.

Regular eye examinations are essential, and any noticeable changes in vision should prompt a visit to your eye care provider. Being proactive about your eye health can significantly reduce the risk of severe complications related to floaters.

How To Heal Floaters

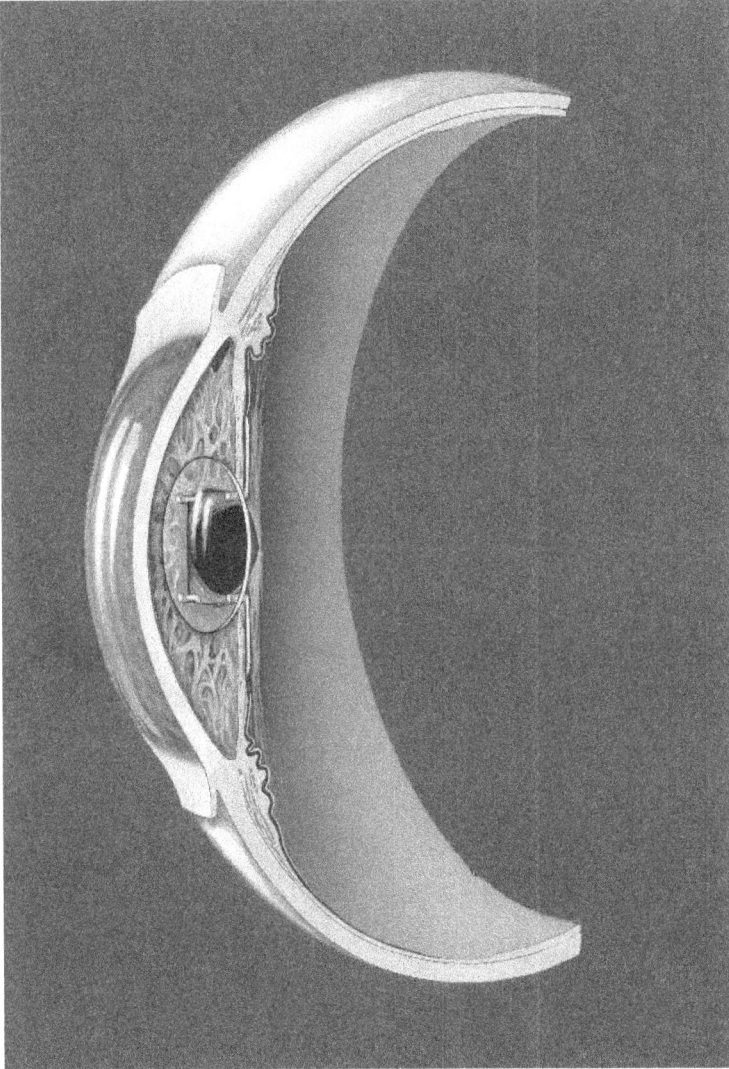

Chapter 2

The Anatomy of the Eye

Structure of the Eye

The eye is a complex organ composed of various structures that work together to facilitate vision. Understanding the anatomy of the eye is essential for individuals concerned about floaters, as these visual disturbances can be related to specific eye conditions. The main components of the eye include the cornea, lens, retina, and vitreous body. Each part plays a critical role in how we perceive the world around us, and any changes or abnormalities in these structures can lead to the development of floaters.

The cornea is the transparent front layer of the eye that allows light to enter. It is responsible for most of the eye's focusing power. Following the cornea, the light passes through the aqueous humor, a clear fluid that helps maintain intraocular pressure and provides nutrients to the eye.

The lens, located behind the iris, fine-tunes the focus of incoming light onto the retina. Changes in the lens, such as those caused by aging or certain eye conditions, can affect visual clarity and may contribute to the perception of floaters.

The retina is a thin layer of tissue located at the back of the eye that converts light into electrical signals, which are then sent to the brain via the optic nerve. It contains specialized cells called photoreceptors, which are crucial for vision.

When floaters occur, they often originate from changes in the vitreous body, a gel-like substance that fills the eye and helps maintain its shape.

As people age, the vitreous can become more liquid, and clumps or strands may form, casting shadows on the retina and creating the appearance of floaters.

The vitreous body is essential for maintaining the eye's structure and stability. It is attached to the retina at various points, and as it shrinks or pulls away from the retina, individuals may experience floaters. While floaters are often harmless, they can sometimes indicate more serious conditions, such as retinal tears or detachments.

Regular eye examinations are crucial for monitoring eye health and identifying any potential issues related to floaters.

In conclusion, understanding the structure of the eye can provide valuable insights for those concerned about floaters. By recognizing how the different components interact and the role they play in vision, individuals can better appreciate the factors that contribute to floaters. This knowledge can empower them to seek appropriate treatments and adopt preventive measures to maintain their eye health.

The Vitreous Humor

The vitreous humor is a clear, gel-like substance that fills the space between the lens and the retina in the eye. Comprising about 80% of the eye's total volume, it plays a crucial role in maintaining the eye's shape and providing support to the retina. The vitreous humor is primarily made up of water, collagen fibers, and hyaluronic acid, which contribute to its unique structure and consistency. Its clarity is essential for allowing light to pass through unobstructed, ensuring that the images we see are sharp and well-defined.

As we age, the vitreous humor undergoes natural changes that can lead to the development of floaters. These floaters are tiny clumps of gel or fibers that cast shadows on the retina, appearing as spots, threads, or cobweb-like structures in our field of vision. While floaters are often harmless, they can become a source of concern for many individuals, particularly if they appear suddenly or are accompanied by flashes of light. Understanding the nature of the vitreous humor and its changes over time can help individuals recognize the normal aging process of the eye and what to expect.

When the vitreous humor begins to shrink and liquefy, it can pull away from the retina, a process known as vitreous detachment. This detachment can lead to an increase in floaters and, in some cases, may pose a risk of retinal tears or detachment. It is important for individuals experiencing new or worsening floaters to seek an eye examination to rule out any serious conditions.

Regular eye check-ups can help monitor the health of the vitreous humor and the retina, ensuring that any issues are addressed promptly.

There are several strategies to support eye health and potentially reduce the impact of floaters. Maintaining a balanced diet rich in antioxidants, omega-3 fatty acids, and vitamins A, C, and E can promote overall eye health. Staying hydrated is also vital, as proper hydration can help maintain the vitreous humor's consistency. Additionally, practicing good eye hygiene, such as taking regular breaks from screens and protecting the eyes from UV rays, can contribute to long-term eye wellness.

While floaters are often a benign aspect of aging, it is essential to be proactive about eye health. Understanding the role of the vitreous humor and its changes can empower individuals to take informed steps toward preserving their vision.

If floaters become bothersome or significantly impact daily life, consulting with an eye care professional for personalized advice and treatment options is recommended. Through awareness and proactive care, individuals can manage their concerns about floaters effectively.

How Floaters Form in the Eye

Floaters are tiny specks, strands, or cobweb-like shapes that drift across your field of vision. They are a common phenomenon, particularly as people age, and understanding how they form in the eye can demystify this often-disconcerting experience. Floaters originate from changes in the vitreous humor, the gel-like substance that fills the eye and helps maintain its shape.

As we age, the vitreous can become more liquid, leading to the collapse of its gel structure. This process creates clumps of collagen fibers, which cast shadows on the retina, the light-sensitive layer at the back of the eye.

The formation of floaters is a natural part of the aging process, but other factors can contribute to their development. Conditions such as myopia, or nearsightedness, can increase the risk of floaters forming. Individuals with a history of eye trauma, inflammation, or previous eye surgeries may also experience a higher prevalence of floaters. Understanding these risk factors can be crucial for individuals who are concerned about their eye health and want to take proactive measures to mitigate the impact of floaters.

In addition to aging and underlying conditions, changes in the vitreous body can also occur due to other factors like dehydration and nutritional deficiencies. The vitreous humor is composed mostly of water, and when the body is dehydrated, the vitreous can shrink, leading to an increase in floaters.

Furthermore, a diet lacking in essential nutrients such as antioxidants, vitamins C and E, and omega-3 fatty acids may affect eye health and the integrity of the vitreous humor. Ensuring adequate hydration and proper nutrition can play a role in maintaining eye health and potentially reducing the formation of floaters.

The appearance of floaters can be alarming, but it is important to recognize that in most cases, they are harmless. However, a sudden increase in floaters or flashes of light can signal more serious conditions, such as retinal detachment or a tear. It is vital for individuals experiencing these symptoms to seek immediate medical attention. Regular eye check-ups can help monitor any changes in vision and ensure that the health of the retina remains intact, allowing for early intervention if necessary.

For those looking to address floaters, understanding their formation is the first step. While floaters are often benign, there are strategies to support overall eye health. These include maintaining a balanced diet rich in eye-friendly nutrients, staying hydrated, and protecting the eyes from excessive stress and strain.

Incorporating practices like eye exercises and mindfulness techniques can also contribute to better eye health. By being informed about how floaters form and implementing preventative measures, individuals can take charge of their eye health and alleviate concerns about floaters.

How To Heal Floaters

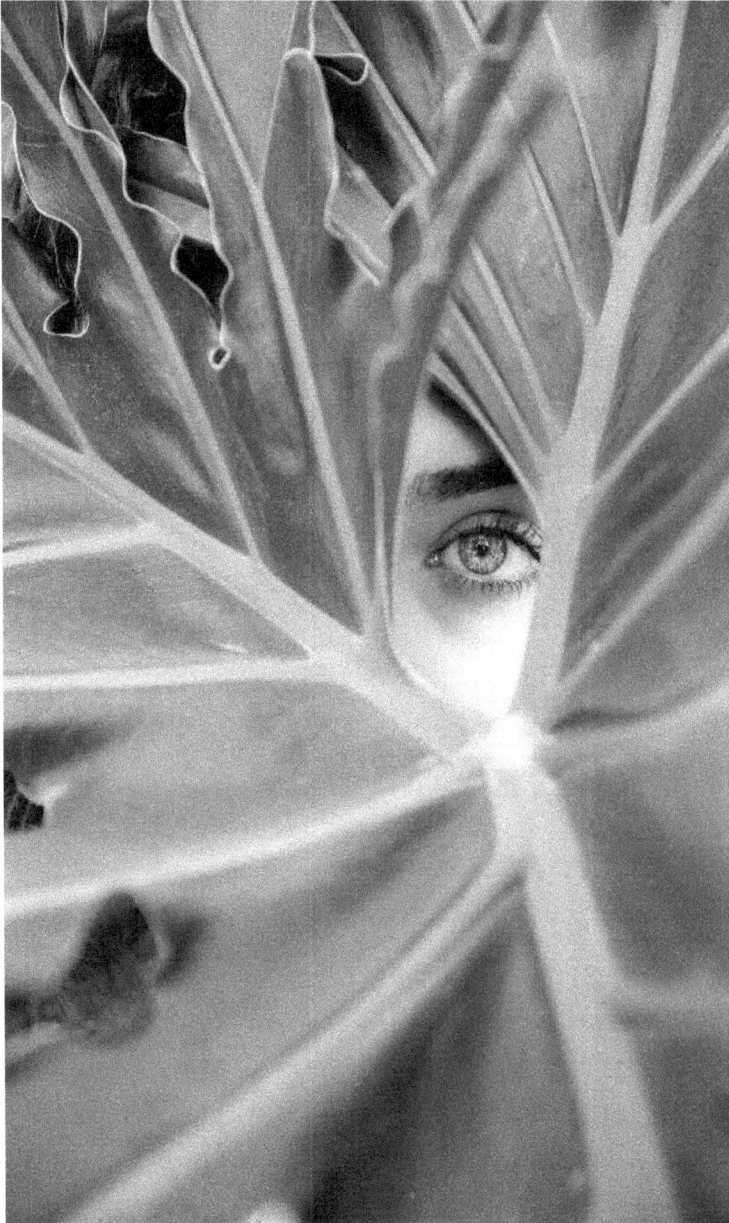

Chapter 3

Assessing Your Floaters

Identifying Symptoms

Identifying symptoms of eye floaters is crucial for anyone concerned about their eye health. Floaters typically appear as small specks, dots, or cobweb-like shapes that drift across the visual field. They are often more noticeable when looking at a plain background, such as a blue sky or a white wall. Understanding the nature of these visual disturbances can help individuals better assess their condition and seek appropriate guidance if necessary.

In addition to the common appearance of floaters, individuals may also experience flashes of light or a sudden increase in the number of floaters. These flashes may occur when the vitreous gel within the eye pulls on the retina, causing a brief sensation of light. While occasional floaters are generally harmless, a sudden increase in floaters or flashes can indicate a more serious issue, such as a retinal tear or detachment, warranting immediate medical attention.

Some individuals might also notice a change in the overall quality of their vision. This could manifest as blurred vision, difficulty focusing, or a shadowy effect in their peripheral vision. These symptoms can be alarming, especially if they develop suddenly.

It is essential to distinguish between benign floaters and symptoms that could suggest a more serious underlying condition, as timely intervention can significantly affect outcomes.

Another symptom worth noting is the emotional and psychological impact of floaters. Many individuals experience anxiety or frustration due to the constant presence of floaters in their vision. This distress can lead to decreased quality of life, as individuals may find it challenging to engage in activities they once enjoyed.

Recognizing this aspect of floaters is important, as managing the emotional response can be part of the healing process.

Finally, keeping a record of symptoms can be beneficial for those concerned about floaters. Note any changes in the frequency, size, or appearance of floaters, as well as any accompanying symptoms like flashes of light or visual disturbances. This information can be invaluable when consulting with an eye care professional, as it provides insight into the progression of the condition and helps guide treatment options. By being proactive and informed, individuals can take significant steps toward managing their eye health effectively.

Self-Assessment Techniques

Self-assessment techniques are essential for individuals concerned about floaters, as they provide a means to evaluate eye health and identify potential changes in vision. Understanding the nature and frequency of floaters can help individuals discern whether they are experiencing normal visual phenomena or if they need to seek professional medical advice. By employing specific self-assessment methods, individuals can gain insights into their eye health and take proactive steps towards managing floaters effectively.

One effective self-assessment technique involves monitoring the frequency and type of floaters experienced. Individuals should take note of when floaters appear, how often they occur, and any patterns that may emerge over time. Keeping a diary can be beneficial; documenting the size, shape, and movement of floaters can help identify whether they are increasing in number or changing in appearance. This information can be crucial when discussing symptoms with an eye care professional, as it provides a clearer picture of the individual's eye health status.

Another technique involves conducting visual tests at home. Simple exercises, such as focusing on a blank surface or a bright light, can help individuals determine if floaters interfere with their vision.

By noting whether floaters obstruct their ability to see clearly or if they diminish under certain conditions, individuals can assess the impact of floaters on their daily activities. This self-evaluation can empower individuals to take necessary actions, such as adjusting lighting or using visual aids, to minimize discomfort caused by floaters.

Additionally, individuals can benefit from assessing their overall eye health through lifestyle evaluation. Factors such as diet, hydration, and screen time play a significant role in eye health. Maintaining a balanced diet rich in nutrients beneficial for eye health, such as vitamins A, C, and E, along with omega-3 fatty acids, can support visual clarity.

Regular breaks from screen time can also reduce eye strain, potentially alleviating the perception of floaters. By integrating these lifestyle assessments into their routine, individuals can foster a healthier environment for their eyes.

Finally, reflecting on any underlying health conditions is crucial for a comprehensive self-assessment. Conditions such as diabetes, hypertension, or autoimmune disorders can affect eye health and contribute to the development of floaters. Individuals should consider their medical history and any medications they are taking, as some can have side effects that impact vision. Engaging in open dialogue with healthcare providers about any concerns or changes in health can lead to better management strategies and improved overall eye health.

By employing these self-assessment techniques, individuals can take informed steps toward understanding and addressing their concerns about floaters.

Keeping a Floaters Diary

Keeping a floaters diary can be an essential tool for individuals concerned about eye floaters. This practice involves documenting your experiences with floaters, including their frequency, size, and any changes in your vision.

By maintaining a detailed record, you can gain insight into your floaters and identify patterns or triggers that may contribute to their occurrence. This information can be invaluable when discussing your condition with healthcare professionals, as it provides a clearer picture of your symptoms and their potential impact on your daily life.

In your floaters diary, include specific details about when you notice the floaters most frequently. Are they more prominent during certain times of the day? Do they seem to increase during activities such as reading or using digital devices?

Noting these factors can help in recognizing environmental influences or lifestyle habits that may exacerbate your floaters. Additionally, documenting any accompanying symptoms, such as headaches or eye strain, can further aid in understanding your overall eye health.

Another important aspect to consider is the emotional impact of floaters. Many individuals experience anxiety or frustration due to their presence. Record your feelings and reactions when floaters appear, as this can help you track how they affect your mental well-being.

Understanding the psychological aspect of living with floaters can guide you in developing coping strategies and may also serve as a discussion point with your eye care provider for more comprehensive treatment options.

As you maintain your diary, it may be beneficial to incorporate other observations related to your eye health. For example, note any changes in vision, the effectiveness of eye exercises, dietary adjustments, or alternative therapies you may be trying.

This holistic approach can provide a more complete understanding of your condition and may highlight connections between various factors impacting your floaters. Over time, this information can contribute to a more personalized strategy for managing and potentially reducing floaters.

Finally, consider sharing your floaters diary with your eye care specialist during check-ups. This documentation can enhance communication between you and your healthcare provider, allowing for a more focused discussion on your symptoms and treatment options.

By actively participating in your eye health management and being proactive about your experiences, you empower yourself in the journey towards healing floaters, equipping yourself with knowledge and insights that can lead to effective strategies for improvement.

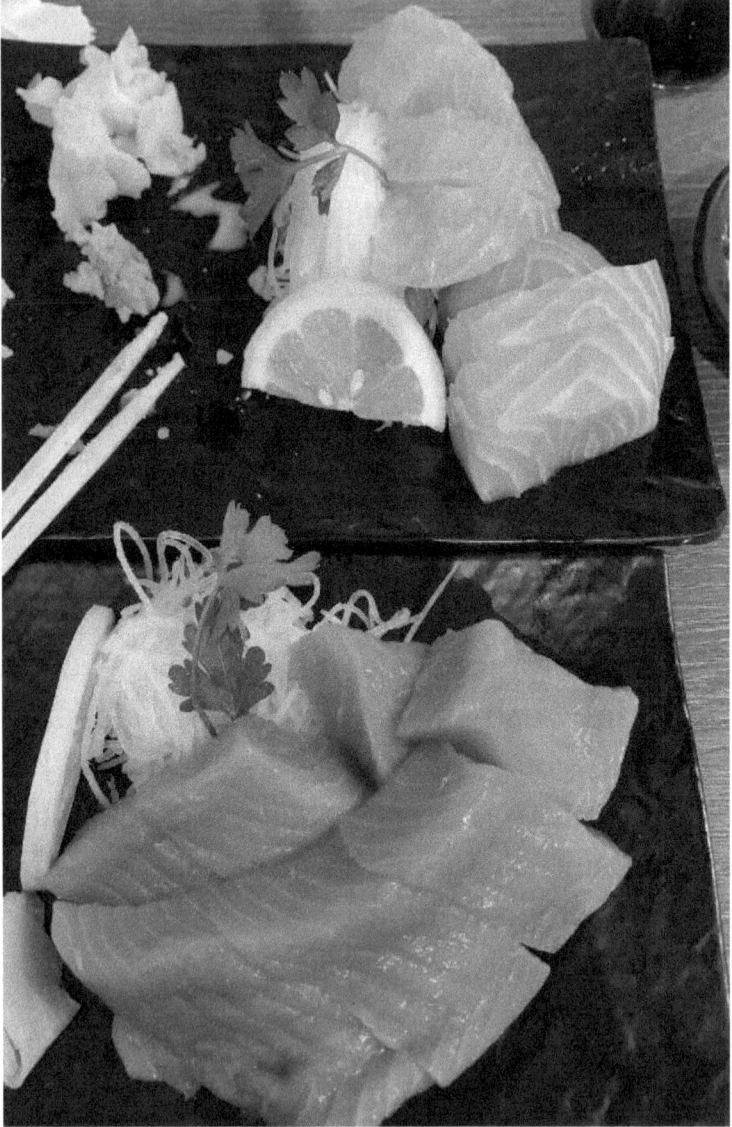

Chapter 4

Lifestyle Changes for Eye Health

Nutrition for Eye Health

Nutrition plays a pivotal role in maintaining optimal eye health and can significantly impact conditions such as floaters. A well-balanced diet rich in essential nutrients supports the overall function of the eyes and can help mitigate the effects of age-related changes.

Key vitamins and minerals, including vitamins A, C, E, and various carotenoids, are crucial for protecting the eyes from oxidative stress and promoting healthy vision.

By incorporating these nutrients into your diet, you can create a foundation for better eye health and potentially alleviate the discomfort associated with floaters.

Vitamin A is essential for maintaining the integrity of the retina and overall eye function. It plays a critical role in the production of rhodopsin, a pigment in the retina that helps you see in low-light conditions. Foods rich in vitamin A, such as carrots, sweet potatoes, and leafy greens, should be integral to your daily meals.

Additionally, beta-carotene, a precursor to vitamin A found in colorful fruits and vegetables, offers potent antioxidant properties that can protect the eyes from harmful free radicals.

Vitamin C is another powerful antioxidant that supports eye health by protecting the lens and retina from oxidative damage. Studies have shown that a diet high in vitamin C may lower the risk of cataracts and age-related macular degeneration, conditions that can exacerbate floaters. Citrus fruits, strawberries, bell peppers, and broccoli are excellent sources of vitamin C. Including these foods in your diet can provide the necessary protection against oxidative stress and enhance overall eye health.

Vitamin E, along with other antioxidants, helps to neutralize free radicals that can damage eye cells. This vitamin is particularly beneficial in reducing the risk of age-related eye diseases. Nuts, seeds, and vegetable oils are rich sources of vitamin E, and incorporating these foods into your snacks and meals can contribute to better eye health.

Additionally, omega-3 fatty acids, found in fatty fish like salmon and flaxseeds, are essential in maintaining the structure and function of cell membranes in the retina, further supporting eye health.

Lastly, staying hydrated is crucial for eye health. Dehydration can lead to dry eyes, which may exacerbate the perception of floaters. Drinking plenty of water and consuming water-rich foods like cucumbers and watermelon can help maintain adequate hydration levels.

By focusing on a diet rich in these vital nutrients and staying hydrated, individuals concerned about floaters can take proactive steps to support their eye health and potentially reduce the occurrence and impact of floaters.

Hydration and Its Importance

Hydration plays a crucial role in maintaining overall health, and its importance cannot be overstated when it comes to eye health, particularly for those concerned about floaters. The human body is composed of approximately 60% water, and every system, including the eyes, relies on adequate hydration to function optimally.

The eyes require a consistent supply of water to maintain their shape and to keep the vitreous humor, the gel-like substance that fills the eye, properly hydrated. When the body is dehydrated, the vitreous can become less viscous, potentially leading to the formation or exacerbation of floaters.

The relationship between hydration and eye health is not just limited to the physical properties of the vitreous humor. Hydration also influences the production of tears, which are vital for maintaining the surface of the eye. Tears help to wash away debris and provide essential nutrients to the cornea.

A well-hydrated body produces an adequate amount of tears, which can reduce eye strain and irritation often associated with floaters. People who experience dry eyes may notice an increase in floaters, as the discomfort can cause them to strain their eyes more, leading to further complications.

To maintain optimal hydration, it is essential to consume an adequate amount of fluids daily. The general recommendation is to drink at least eight 8-ounce glasses of water, though individual needs may vary based on factors such as activity level, climate, and overall health.

Additionally, incorporating hydrating foods, such as fruits and vegetables, into your diet can contribute to your daily fluid intake. Foods like cucumbers, oranges, and watermelon not only provide hydration but also contain vitamins and antioxidants that support eye health.

Furthermore, it is important to be mindful of substances that can lead to dehydration. Caffeine and alcohol, for instance, have diuretic effects that can increase fluid loss in the body.

If consumed in excess, these beverages can lead to dehydration, negatively impacting not only general health but also eye health. Balancing these drinks with ample water intake can help mitigate their dehydrating effects, ensuring that your body and eyes remain adequately hydrated.

In conclusion, prioritizing hydration is a simple yet effective strategy for supporting eye health and potentially alleviating concerns related to floaters. By ensuring that you drink enough water and consume hydrating foods, you can help keep your eyes functioning smoothly.

As part of a comprehensive approach to managing floaters, maintaining proper hydration should be a fundamental consideration for anyone looking to improve their eye health and overall well-being.

The Role of Exercise

Exercise plays a crucial role in maintaining overall eye health and can be particularly beneficial for those concerned about floaters. Regular physical activity enhances blood circulation, which is vital for the health of the retina and other eye structures. Improved circulation ensures that the eyes receive a consistent supply of oxygen and nutrients, promoting optimal function and potentially reducing the occurrences of floaters.

Furthermore, exercise can help manage systemic health issues such as diabetes and hypertension, which are known risk factors for vision problems.

Engaging in aerobic exercises, such as brisk walking, jogging, or cycling, can significantly contribute to cardiovascular health. These activities increase heart rate and blood flow, fostering a healthier environment for the eyes. Additionally, aerobic exercises stimulate the release of endorphins, which can alleviate stress and anxiety.

Stress is known to impact overall health, including eye health, making it imperative to incorporate stress-reducing activities into one's routine. By managing stress through physical activity, individuals may find a reduction in the perception of floaters.

Strength training is another important aspect of an exercise regimen that can benefit eye health. Building muscle strength supports better posture and alignment, which can relieve strain on the eyes and surrounding muscles. Poor posture may lead to eye fatigue and discomfort, exacerbating the perception of floaters. Incorporating strength training exercises, such as weightlifting or resistance band workouts, can create a well-rounded fitness program that enhances not only physical strength but also overall eye comfort.

Flexibility and balance exercises, such as yoga or tai chi, offer additional benefits for eye health. These practices encourage mindful movement and help improve coordination and spatial awareness. Yoga, in particular, incorporates specific poses and breathing techniques that can enhance blood flow and oxygenation to the eyes. Furthermore, the meditative aspects of these exercises can promote relaxation, further reducing stress levels.

This combination of physical and mental benefits makes flexibility and balance exercises an excellent addition to any routine focused on improving eye health.

It is essential to approach exercise with consistency and mindfulness. Individuals concerned about floaters should aim for a balanced exercise regimen that includes aerobic, strength, and flexibility training. Consulting with a healthcare professional before starting any new exercise program is advisable, especially for those with pre-existing conditions or those who have been sedentary.

By integrating regular exercise into daily life, individuals can not only enhance their overall well-being but also support their eye health and potentially mitigate the impact of floaters.

How To Heal Floaters

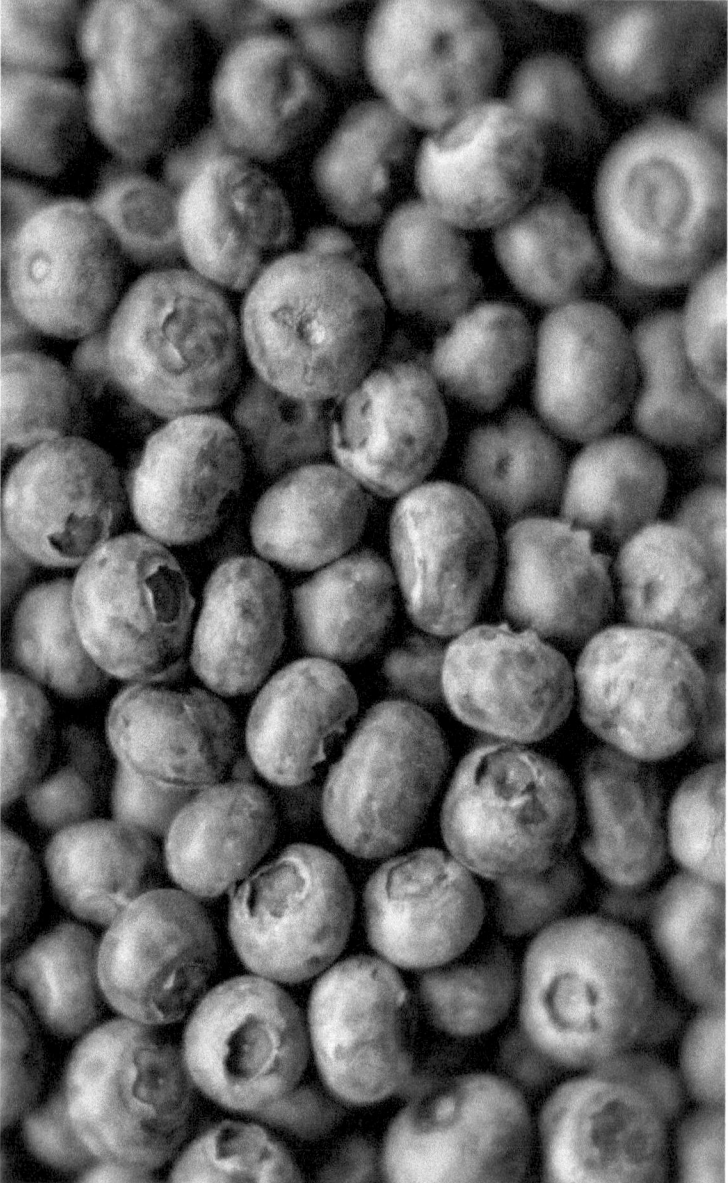

Chapter 5

Natural Remedies for Floaters

Herbal Supplements

Herbal supplements have gained attention in recent years as a potential aid for various health issues, including eye health. For those concerned about floaters, exploring herbal remedies may offer additional support alongside traditional treatments.

Many herbs are known for their antioxidant properties, which can be beneficial in combating oxidative stress in the eyes. Herbs such as bilberry, ginkgo biloba, and eyebright have been traditionally used to support vision and eye health, making them worth considering for individuals seeking natural alternatives.

Bilberry is often highlighted for its rich content of anthocyanins, powerful antioxidants that may help improve blood circulation and enhance night vision. This herb has been studied for its effects on retinal health, and some preliminary research suggests that it may aid in reducing the risk of age-related eye issues.

Incorporating bilberry extract into your daily routine could potentially provide benefits not only for general eye health but also for managing floaters.

Ginkgo biloba is another herb that has been used for centuries to support cognitive function and circulation. Its potential benefits for eye health stem from its ability to improve blood flow, which is crucial for delivering essential nutrients and oxygen to the eyes.

Some studies have indicated that ginkgo biloba may help alleviate symptoms related to visual disturbances. For individuals dealing with floaters, enhancing circulation through this supplement might contribute positively to overall eye wellness.

Eyebright is a lesser-known herb but has been traditionally used to treat various eye conditions. It contains compounds believed to have anti-inflammatory and astringent properties, which may help soothe irritated eyes. While specific studies on its effectiveness for floaters are limited, its historical use in herbal medicine suggests that it could be beneficial for those experiencing discomfort. Eyebright can be consumed in tea form or as a supplement, providing a gentle approach to supporting eye health.

While herbal supplements can offer potential advantages, it is essential to approach their use with caution. Consulting with a healthcare professional before adding any new supplement to your regimen is crucial, especially for individuals with pre-existing health conditions or those taking medications.

Additionally, herbal remedies should be viewed as complementary to a comprehensive eye health strategy that includes proper nutrition, regular eye examinations, and lifestyle modifications. By integrating herbal supplements thoughtfully, individuals concerned about floaters may find a holistic approach to enhancing their eye health.

Essential Oils

Essential oils have gained popularity in holistic health practices, offering various therapeutic benefits that can support overall well-being, including eye health. These concentrated plant extracts contain potent properties that can help alleviate discomfort and promote a sense of relaxation. For individuals concerned about eye floaters, integrating essential oils into their daily routine may provide additional support for eye health and contribute to a more balanced state of being.

One of the most commonly recommended essential oils for eye care is lavender oil. Known for its calming and soothing properties, lavender oil can help reduce stress and anxiety, which may indirectly benefit eye health. Stress can exacerbate the perception of floaters, so incorporating lavender oil into a relaxation routine, perhaps through diffusing it in the home or using it in a calming massage, may help ease overall tension. Additionally, lavender oil possesses antioxidant properties, which can assist in combating oxidative stress within the body, potentially benefiting the eyes.

Another essential oil worth considering is chamomile. This oil is renowned for its anti-inflammatory and soothing effects, making it a suitable choice for those experiencing discomfort associated with floaters. Chamomile can be used in a warm compress applied to the closed eyelids to promote relaxation and reduce inflammation.

Its gentle properties make it a safe option for individuals looking to alleviate symptoms without harsh chemicals, fostering a natural approach to eye care.

Frankincense oil is also notable for its potential benefits to eye health. This oil has been traditionally used for its anti-inflammatory and healing properties. When diluted with a carrier oil, frankincense can be gently massaged around the eye area, promoting circulation and potentially aiding in the nourishment of eye tissues.

While caution should always be exercised with essential oils near the eyes, frankincense offers a promising avenue for those exploring natural remedies for floaters.

It is essential to approach the use of essential oils with knowledge and care. Always ensure that oils are properly diluted before application, especially around sensitive areas such as the eyes. Consulting with a healthcare professional or an experienced aromatherapist can provide guidance tailored to individual needs and concerns. By incorporating essential oils into a holistic health strategy, individuals concerned about floaters may find additional support in their journey toward improved eye health.

Homeopathy

Homeopathy is a holistic approach to healing that focuses on treating the individual as a whole rather than just addressing specific symptoms. In the context of managing eye floaters, homeopathy can offer a unique perspective and potential benefits. This approach is based on the principle of "like cures like," meaning that substances that produce symptoms in a healthy person can be used in diluted forms to treat similar symptoms in someone who is ill. For those experiencing floaters, homeopathic remedies may help alleviate the discomfort and improve overall eye health.

Several homeopathic remedies are commonly suggested for individuals concerned about floaters. For instance, remedies such as Pulsatilla and Silicea have been noted for their effectiveness in treating visual disturbances. Pulsatilla is often recommended for patients who experience floaters accompanied by emotional upset, while Silicea may be beneficial for those who have a history of eye issues or general weakness.

It is essential to consult a qualified homeopath to determine the most appropriate remedy based on individual symptoms and overall health.

Another important aspect of homeopathy is the individualized treatment plan it promotes. Unlike conventional medicine, which often prescribes a one-size-fits-all solution, homeopathy emphasizes tailored remedies. A homeopath will consider your constitution, lifestyle, and specific symptoms before recommending a treatment. This personalized approach can help address the underlying causes of floaters rather than merely masking the symptoms, potentially leading to more effective long-term relief.

In addition to specific remedies, lifestyle factors play a crucial role in homeopathic treatment. Homeopaths often encourage patients to adopt healthy habits that support eye health. This may include dietary changes, stress management techniques, and exercises aimed at improving overall well-being. By integrating these lifestyle modifications with homeopathic remedies, individuals can enhance the effectiveness of their treatment and promote better eye health.

While many people have reported positive outcomes with homeopathy for floaters, it is important to approach this treatment modality with realistic expectations. Homeopathy may not work for everyone, and its efficacy can vary depending on the individual.

It is advisable to combine homeopathic treatment with other evidence-based practices for eye health, such as regular eye exams and proper nutrition. By doing so, individuals can create a comprehensive strategy for managing floaters and maintaining optimal eye health.

How To Heal Floaters

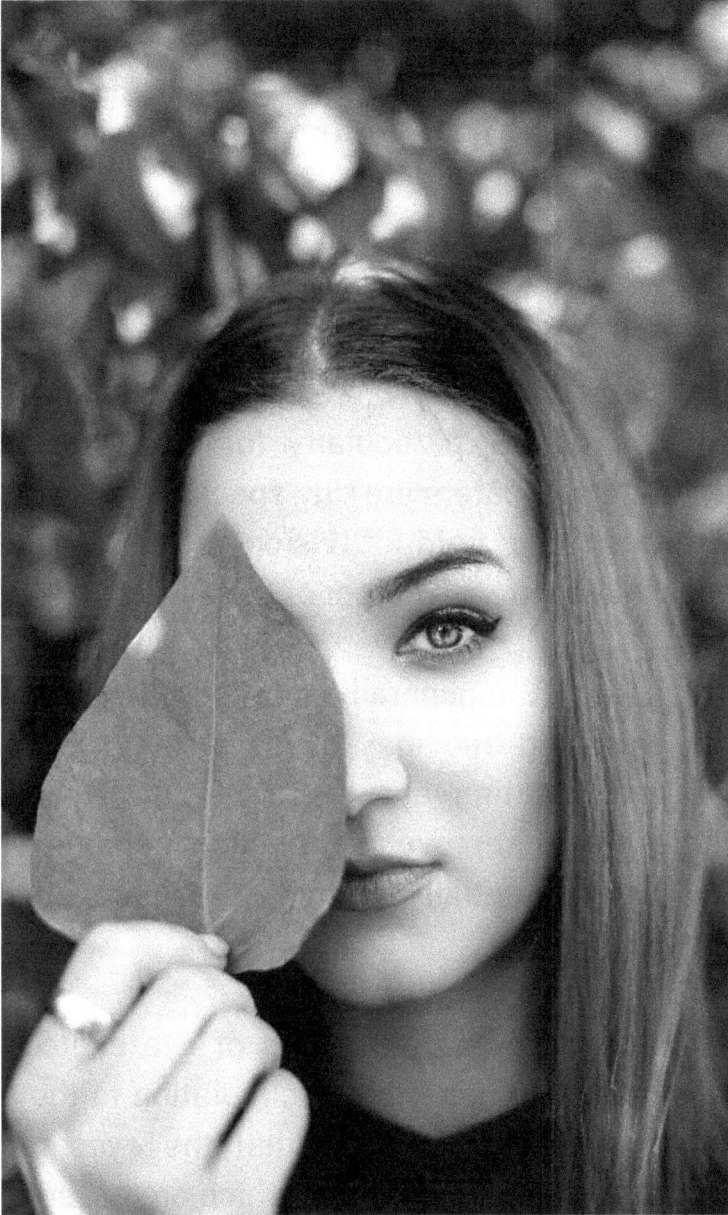

Chapter 6
Eye Exercises

Importance of Eye Exercises

Eye exercises play a crucial role in maintaining overall eye health, particularly for those concerned about floaters. Floaters are tiny specks or threads that drift through the field of vision, often caused by changes in the vitreous humor of the eye.

While they are generally harmless, their presence can be annoying and may cause anxiety about eye health. Incorporating eye exercises into your daily routine can help improve eye function, enhance visual clarity, and potentially reduce the perception of floaters.

One of the primary benefits of eye exercises is that they promote better blood circulation to the eyes. Improved circulation ensures that the eyes receive adequate nutrients and oxygen, which are essential for optimal function.

This can be particularly beneficial for those experiencing floaters, as the health of the vitreous humor and surrounding structures can be directly influenced by proper blood flow. Eye exercises such as focusing on distant and near objects can stimulate the muscles around the eyes, enhancing their flexibility and reducing strain.

Eye exercises can also aid in reducing eye strain, which is often exacerbated by prolonged screen time and insufficient breaks. When the eyes are overworked, they can become fatigued, leading to increased visibility of floaters.

Regularly practicing exercises such as palming, where you gently cover your eyes with your palms to relax them, can help alleviate this strain. By allowing the eyes to rest and recover, you may notice a decrease in the discomfort associated with floaters.

Additionally, eye exercises can improve visual acuity and coordination. Engaging in activities that require tracking moving objects can strengthen the eye muscles and enhance focus. This can be particularly useful for individuals who find that floaters distract them from their visual tasks.

Improving coordination between the eyes can lead to a more stable and clear visual field, making floaters less intrusive in daily life.

Incorporating eye exercises into a daily routine can be a simple yet effective strategy for managing floaters. These exercises can be performed anywhere and at any time, making them an accessible option for those looking to improve their eye health. By dedicating just a few minutes each day to eye exercises, individuals can take proactive steps toward enhancing their visual well-being, potentially minimizing the impact of floaters on their lives.

Basic Eye Exercises

Basic eye exercises can play a significant role in maintaining eye health and possibly alleviating the discomfort caused by floaters. These exercises are designed to strengthen the eye muscles, improve circulation, and enhance overall visual function. Incorporating a routine of eye exercises can be beneficial for individuals looking to reduce the impact of floaters and improve their visual clarity.

One effective exercise is the "Palming" technique. To perform this exercise, sit comfortably and rub your palms together to generate warmth. Once warm, gently cup your palms over your closed eyes without applying pressure.

This technique allows your eyes to relax and can help relieve tension that may contribute to visual disturbances. Hold this position for a few minutes, focusing on your breathing, and visualize a calming image to enhance relaxation.

Another beneficial exercise is the "Focus Shift." Begin by holding your finger or a small object about six inches from your face. Focus on it for a few seconds, then shift your gaze to an object in the distance, ideally about 20 feet away.

Hold your focus on the distant object for a few seconds before returning your gaze to your finger. This exercise helps to improve the flexibility of the eye muscles and can enhance your ability to switch focus, which is essential for clear vision.

The "Eye Rolling" exercise is also advantageous for eye health. To perform this exercise, sit comfortably and close your eyes. Slowly roll your eyes in a circular motion, first clockwise and then counterclockwise. This movement helps to increase blood flow to the eyes and can relieve eye strain. Repeat this exercise for about 30 seconds in each direction to maximize its benefits.

Lastly, practicing "Near and Far Focus" can help strengthen your eye muscles. For this exercise, hold a small object close to your face and focus on it for a few seconds. Then, switch your gaze to a distant object. Alternate between the two for several minutes.

This exercise encourages the eye muscles to work together, improving their coordination and flexibility, which may contribute to a reduction in the perception of floaters over time. Regularly incorporating these exercises into your daily routine can support eye health and potentially ease the discomfort associated with floaters.

Advanced Techniques

Advanced techniques for managing and potentially alleviating eye floaters involve a combination of lifestyle changes, dietary adjustments, and professional interventions. As individuals become more aware of their eye health, they seek effective strategies beyond basic remedies. These advanced techniques can empower those concerned about floaters to take proactive steps in their healing journey.

One significant approach is the incorporation of specific eye exercises into daily routines. Eye exercises, such as the 20-20-20 rule, encourage individuals to take breaks from screens every 20 minutes by looking at something 20 feet away for 20 seconds. This practice helps alleviate eye strain, which can contribute to the perception of floaters.

Additionally, exercises that involve moving the eyes in various directions can promote better circulation and overall eye health. Techniques such as focusing on near and far objects can strengthen the eye muscles and may reduce the prominence of floaters over time.

Nutrition plays a crucial role in eye health, and certain dietary adjustments can be beneficial for those looking to manage floaters. Foods rich in antioxidants, such as leafy greens, berries, and fish high in omega-3 fatty acids, support overall eye function and may help in maintaining the health of the vitreous gel in the eye.

Supplements like lutein and zeaxanthin are known to promote retinal health and can be an effective addition to one's diet. Hydration is equally important; ensuring adequate water intake helps maintain the viscosity of the vitreous fluid, potentially minimizing the occurrence of floaters.

For those seeking more immediate solutions, professional interventions may offer advanced options. Laser treatment, known as YAG laser vitreolysis, is a procedure where a laser is used to break down floaters, making them less noticeable. This minimally invasive technique requires a skilled ophthalmologist and can provide significant relief for individuals with bothersome floaters.

Another option includes vitrectomy, a more invasive procedure that removes the vitreous gel entirely, along with the floaters. While effective, vitrectomy carries potential risks and is typically reserved for severe cases where floaters significantly impair vision.

Finally, maintaining regular eye check-ups is essential for anyone concerned about floaters. Eye health can change over time, and routine examinations allow for early detection of any underlying issues that may contribute to floaters. An eye care professional can provide personalized recommendations and monitor the progress of any techniques employed.

By combining advanced techniques such as eye exercises, dietary improvements, professional treatments, and regular check-ups, individuals can take meaningful steps toward managing floaters and enhancing their overall eye health.

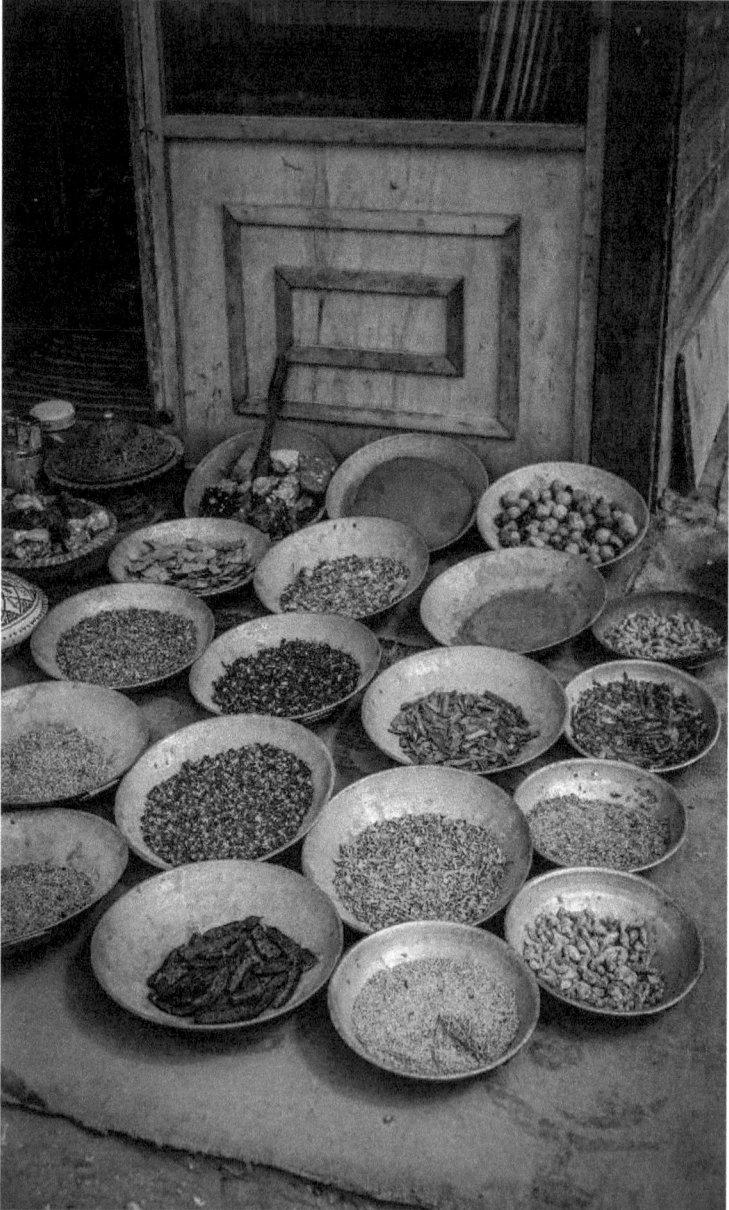

Chapter 7
Medical Treatments

Laser Therapy

Laser therapy is an innovative approach to managing eye floaters, which are often perceived as small specks or threads drifting across one's field of vision. This treatment utilizes a specific type of laser, known as YAG (yttrium-aluminum-garnet) laser, to target and break apart the floaters within the vitreous humor of the eye.

The procedure aims to reduce the visibility of floaters, offering relief to individuals who find them distracting or bothersome. While laser therapy is not suitable for everyone, it has shown promise for certain patients, particularly those with significant floaters that interfere with daily activities.

During a laser therapy session, patients are typically positioned comfortably in a chair, and the procedure is performed in an outpatient setting. A local anesthetic may be administered to minimize discomfort during the treatment. The doctor will use a specialized lens to focus the laser on the floaters.

The energy from the laser effectively vaporizes the floaters or breaks them into smaller pieces, which can then be absorbed by the body or drift out of the patient's line of sight. The entire process usually takes less than an hour, making it a relatively quick and efficient option for those seeking relief from floaters.

While laser therapy can be beneficial, it is essential for patients to discuss their specific conditions with an eye care professional. Not all types of floaters may respond well to laser treatment. For instance, floaters that are large or dense may require additional sessions or may not respond effectively to the laser. Furthermore, potential risks associated with the procedure, such as retinal damage or increased intraocular pressure, should be thoroughly evaluated. A qualified ophthalmologist will conduct a comprehensive eye examination to determine if laser therapy is an appropriate treatment option.

The success rate of laser therapy for floaters can vary among individuals. Some patients report a significant reduction in the prominence of their floaters, leading to improved visual quality and comfort. Others may experience little to no change. It is crucial for patients to have realistic expectations before undergoing the procedure.

Additionally, while laser therapy may alleviate floaters, it does not prevent new floaters from forming in the future, which is an important consideration for individuals with a history of floaters.

In conclusion, laser therapy represents a modern treatment option for individuals concerned about eye floaters. As with any medical procedure, it is vital to weigh the benefits against the potential risks and to seek advice from an experienced eye care professional.

For those who find floaters to be a disruptive element in their visual experience, exploring laser therapy as part of a comprehensive management plan may lead to effective relief and a return to clearer, more comfortable vision.

Vitrectomy

Vitrectomy is a surgical procedure that involves the removal of the vitreous gel from the eye, which can be a potential option for individuals experiencing significant floaters. This procedure is typically considered when floaters become disruptive to daily activities or when they interfere with vision to a degree that impacts quality of life. While floaters are often harmless and a natural part of the aging process, in some cases, they can indicate underlying issues, such as retinal tears or detachment. Thus, consulting with an eye specialist to determine the necessity of vitrectomy is essential.

The procedure itself involves the surgeon making small incisions in the eye to access the vitreous cavity. The vitreous gel is then carefully removed, allowing the surgeon to examine the retina for any abnormalities. In many cases, this step also allows for the treatment of any concurrent conditions, such as repairing a retinal tear. Following the removal of the vitreous, the cavity may be filled with a saline solution, gas bubble, or silicone oil to help maintain the eye's shape and support the retina during the healing process.

While vitrectomy can provide immediate relief from floaters, it is important to consider the associated risks. As with any surgical procedure, complications can arise, including infection, bleeding, or even changes in vision. Moreover, not all patients experience complete resolution of floaters post-surgery. In some instances, new floaters may develop after the procedure due to changes in the eye's structure. Therefore, it is vital to weigh the potential benefits against the risks with a qualified ophthalmologist.

Recovery from vitrectomy generally involves a period of monitoring and follow-up appointments to ensure proper healing. Patients may be advised to avoid certain activities that could strain the eye, such as heavy lifting or vigorous exercise, during the initial recovery phase.

Additionally, regular eye examinations will help track any changes in vision and ensure that the retina remains healthy. This recovery period allows the eye to adjust to the absence of the vitreous gel and can lead to a gradual improvement in visual clarity.

In conclusion, vitrectomy can be an effective option for those suffering from debilitating floaters, but it is not without its considerations. Individuals contemplating this procedure should engage in thorough discussions with their eye care professionals to understand the implications fully. Exploring all available options and understanding the nature of their floaters will empower patients to make informed decisions about their eye health.

Alternative Medical Approaches

Alternative medical approaches for addressing eye floaters encompass a variety of practices and therapies that aim to promote ocular health and potentially reduce the occurrence of these visual disturbances. While conventional medicine often focuses on observation and reassurance, many individuals seek supplementary methods that may offer relief or improvement.

This subchapter explores several alternative strategies, including dietary adjustments, herbal remedies, acupuncture, and mindfulness practices, all of which may contribute to better eye health and the management of floaters.

Dietary modifications can play a crucial role in eye health. A diet rich in antioxidants, vitamins, and minerals is essential for maintaining the health of the retina and vitreous humor. Foods high in vitamins A, C, and E, as well as omega-3 fatty acids, can support overall eye function. Incorporating leafy greens, colorful fruits, nuts, and fatty fish into daily meals may help reduce oxidative stress in the eyes.

Additionally, staying hydrated is vital, as proper hydration supports the vitreous humor's consistency, potentially minimizing the appearance of floaters.

Herbal remedies have garnered attention for their potential benefits in eye health. Certain herbs, such as bilberry and ginkgo biloba, are believed to enhance circulation and promote retinal health. Bilberry, in particular, is rich in anthocyanins, which may help strengthen blood vessels and improve night vision. Ginkgo biloba is often used for its purported ability to increase blood flow to the eyes, possibly aiding in the management of floaters. It is important for individuals to consult with a healthcare professional before beginning any herbal supplement to ensure safety and efficacy.

Acupuncture is another alternative approach that has gained popularity for its holistic benefits. This traditional Chinese medicine technique involves inserting thin needles into specific points on the body to promote energy flow and balance. Some practitioners suggest that acupuncture may help alleviate symptoms related to floaters by improving blood circulation to the eyes and reducing tension in the surrounding muscles.

While scientific evidence supporting its effectiveness for floaters is limited, many individuals report feeling more relaxed and balanced after treatments, which could indirectly benefit eye health.

Mindfulness and stress reduction techniques can also play a significant role in managing floaters. Practices such as meditation, yoga, and deep breathing exercises may not only enhance mental well-being but can also support physical health. Stress has been associated with various health issues, including eye strain and fatigue, which could potentially exacerbate the perception of floaters.

By adopting a regular mindfulness practice, individuals can foster a sense of calm and focus, which may help them cope better with the visual disturbances caused by floaters. Integrating these alternative medical approaches into a comprehensive eye care regimen can empower individuals to take proactive steps towards their eye health.

How To Heal Floaters

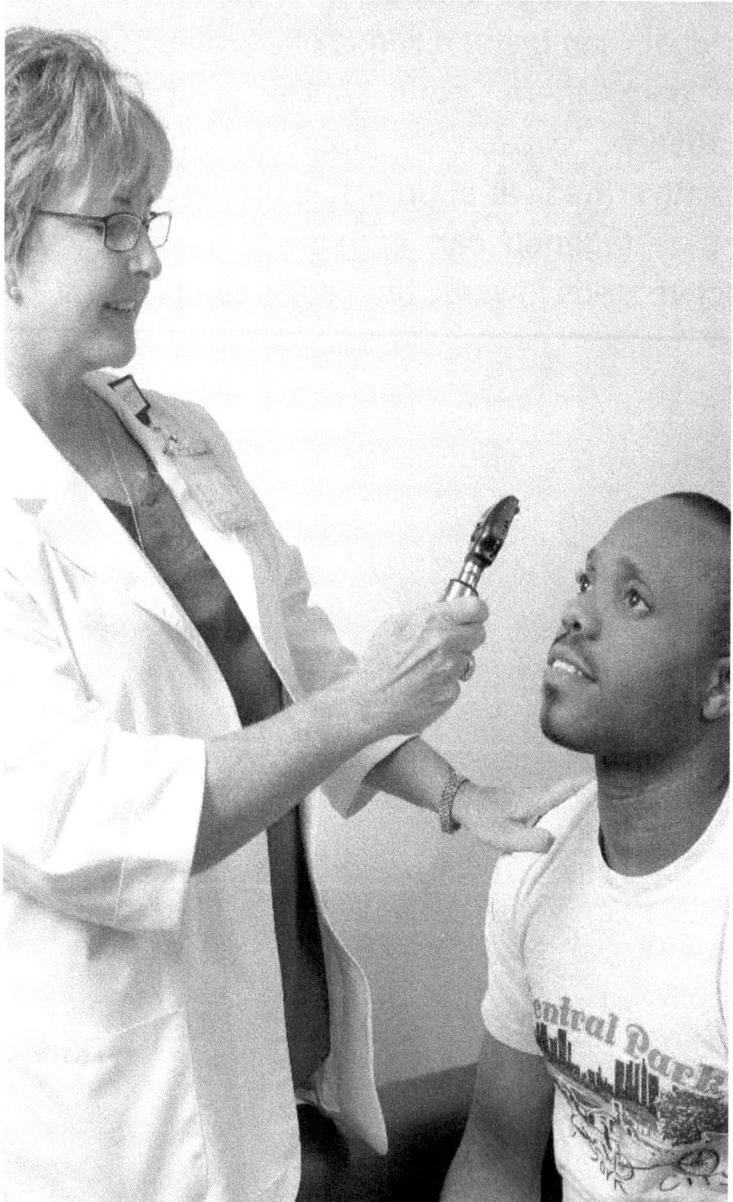

Chapter 8
Preventive Strategies

Regular Eye Check-Ups

Regular eye check-ups are a crucial aspect of maintaining overall eye health, particularly for individuals concerned about floaters. Floaters, which appear as small specks, shadows, or cobweb-like shapes in the field of vision, can be a common occurrence, especially as one ages. However, they can also indicate underlying eye conditions that may require attention. By scheduling routine eye examinations, individuals can not only monitor the presence of floaters but also ensure that their eyes remain in optimal condition.

During an eye check-up, an eye care professional will conduct a comprehensive evaluation of the eyes. This typically includes a visual acuity test, which measures how well one can see at various distances, and a dilated eye exam, where eye drops are used to widen the pupils.

This allows the doctor to thoroughly examine the retina and vitreous for any signs of abnormalities. Regular check-ups help in early detection of potential issues such as retinal tears or detachments, which can be serious complications associated with floaters.

Moreover, eye check-ups serve as an opportunity for individuals to discuss their specific concerns regarding floaters with their eye care provider. Patients can ask questions about the nature of their floaters, any changes they may have noticed, and whether these changes warrant further investigation. Open communication during these visits can lead to a better understanding of the condition and its implications, empowering individuals to make informed decisions about their eye health.

In addition to monitoring floaters, regular eye exams can help identify other health issues that may impact vision. Conditions such as diabetes and hypertension can manifest through changes in the eyes, and early detection through routine check-ups can lead to timely intervention. Maintaining a regular schedule of eye examinations not only aids in managing floaters but also contributes to the overall health of the eyes and the body.

Lastly, it is essential to emphasize that the frequency of eye check-ups may vary depending on individual risk factors and age. For those experiencing floaters for the first time or noticing a sudden increase in their number, it is advisable to seek an eye examination promptly.

Generally, adults should aim for a comprehensive eye exam every one to two years, but those with existing eye conditions or risk factors might need to visit their eye care professional more frequently. Prioritizing regular eye check-ups is a vital step in the proactive management of floaters and overall eye health.

Protecting Your Eyes from Harm

Protecting your eyes from harm is essential for maintaining overall eye health and preventing conditions that could exacerbate floaters. One of the most significant threats to your eyes comes from harmful UV rays.

Prolonged exposure to sunlight can lead to various eye problems, including cataracts and macular degeneration, which may intensify the perception of floaters. Wearing sunglasses that block 100% of UVA and UVB rays is crucial when outdoors, even on cloudy days, as UV rays can penetrate through clouds. Additionally, consider wearing a wide-brimmed hat for added protection.

Another important aspect of eye safety is minimizing digital eye strain, which has become increasingly prevalent in our technology-driven world. Prolonged screen time can lead to discomfort, fatigue, and blurred vision, potentially worsening the symptoms associated with floaters.

To combat this, adopt the 20-20-20 rule: every 20 minutes, take a 20-second break and focus on something at least 20 feet away. This simple practice helps to relax the eye muscles and reduce strain. Furthermore, ensure your screen is properly adjusted in terms of brightness and contrast to create a comfortable viewing experience.

Nutrition plays a vital role in eye health, and certain dietary choices can help protect your eyes from harm. Foods rich in antioxidants, vitamins C and E, and omega-3 fatty acids can support retinal health and may help reduce the risk of conditions that could contribute to floaters. Leafy greens, carrots, fish, nuts, and citrus fruits are excellent additions to your diet.

Staying hydrated is equally important, as dehydration can lead to dry eyes and discomfort. Aim to drink plenty of water throughout the day to maintain optimal moisture levels in your eyes.

In addition to dietary measures, regular eye examinations are crucial for early detection and prevention of eye issues. Eye care professionals can identify changes in your vision and provide guidance on how to manage floaters effectively.

It is advisable to schedule comprehensive eye exams at least once a year, especially if you notice any sudden changes in your floaters or overall vision. Early intervention can often prevent further complications and help you maintain better eye health.

Lastly, protecting your eyes from physical harm is essential, particularly in environments where injuries could occur. Wearing protective eyewear during activities like sports, home improvement projects, or when exposed to hazardous materials can significantly reduce the risk of eye injuries. Additionally, be mindful of your surroundings, and avoid exposing your eyes to irritants such as smoke, dust, and chemicals. By taking these proactive steps, you can help safeguard your eyes from harm and support your journey toward managing floaters effectively.

Managing Eye Strain

Managing eye strain is a crucial aspect for those concerned about floaters, as excessive strain can exacerbate visual disturbances and discomfort. Eye strain, also known as asthenopia, often arises from prolonged screen time, inadequate lighting, or improper viewing distances. Individuals experiencing floaters may find that their symptoms become more pronounced during periods of intense visual focus. Therefore, understanding and implementing strategies to manage eye strain can play a significant role in maintaining overall eye health.

One effective strategy for managing eye strain is the 20-20-20 rule. This guideline suggests that for every 20 minutes spent looking at a screen or focusing on a task, one should take a 20-second break and look at something 20 feet away.

This practice allows the eye muscles to relax and reduces fatigue. Additionally, incorporating regular breaks into your routine can help alleviate discomfort associated with floaters, as it provides the eyes with necessary respite from constant focus.

Proper lighting also plays a vital role in reducing eye strain. Working in environments with harsh or dim lighting can increase the likelihood of straining the eyes. To minimize strain, ensure that your workspace is well-lit with soft, ambient lighting.

Avoid glare by positioning screens away from windows and using anti-glare screens when necessary. Adequate lighting not only helps in reducing eye fatigue but also contributes to a more comfortable visual experience, which is essential for those coping with floaters.

Moreover, optimizing your screen settings can significantly affect eye comfort. Adjusting the brightness and contrast of your digital devices to match the surrounding light can minimize strain. Using larger text sizes and high-resolution displays can also reduce the effort your eyes need to exert when reading.

For individuals concerned about floaters, these adjustments can create a more soothing environment, allowing for easier visual processing without exacerbating existing symptoms.

Finally, incorporating eye exercises into your daily routine can serve as a proactive measure against eye strain. Simple exercises, such as rolling your eyes, blinking frequently, or practicing the palming technique, can help relax the eye muscles and improve circulation. These exercises can be particularly beneficial for those with floaters, as they promote overall eye health and potentially reduce the frequency and intensity of floaters. By managing eye strain effectively, individuals can create a more comfortable visual experience and support their journey toward better eye health.

How To Heal Floaters

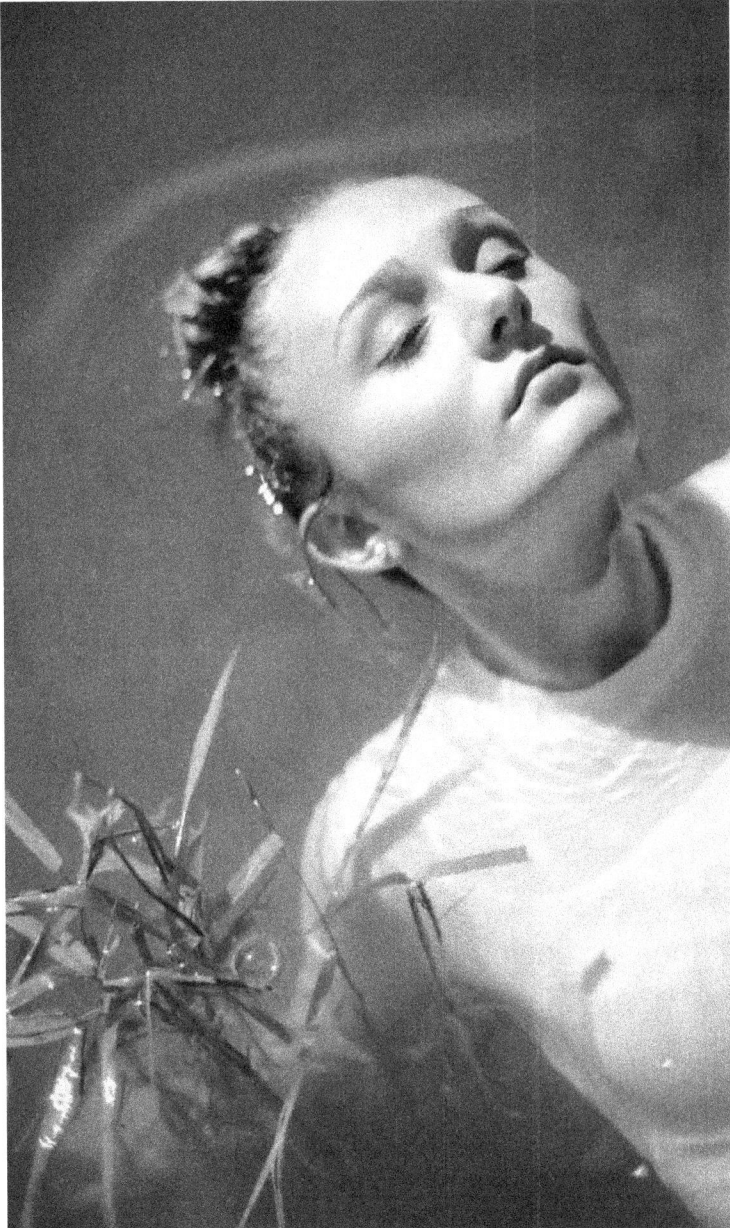

Chapter 9

Coping with Floaters

Emotional and Psychological Impact

The presence of floaters can lead to significant emotional distress and psychological impact for many individuals. Floaters, which are small spots or strands that drift through the field of vision, can be a source of anxiety and frustration. Those who experience this phenomenon often find themselves preoccupied with the condition, leading to heightened levels of stress.

This stress can manifest in various forms, including irritability, difficulty concentrating, and even avoidance of social situations where vision clarity is essential. Understanding these emotional responses is crucial in addressing the overall well-being of individuals coping with floaters.

Anxiety surrounding floaters often stems from a fear of potential underlying eye conditions. Many individuals worry that floaters could signify a more serious issue, such as retinal detachment or other vision-threatening diseases. This fear can exacerbate feelings of helplessness and insecurity, creating a cycle of anxiety that may lead to excessive monitoring of one's vision or obsessive research about the condition. The constant vigilance can take a toll on mental health, with individuals feeling trapped in a loop of worry that can overshadow other aspects of their lives.

Depression can also be a consequence of living with floaters. The persistent visual disturbances can diminish a person's quality of life, impacting their ability to engage in daily activities and enjoy hobbies. This limitation can lead to feelings of isolation and sadness.

For some, the inability to fully participate in life due to floaters can result in a sense of loss and grief for the activities they once loved. Recognizing the link between floaters and depressive symptoms is vital for encouraging those affected to seek support and explore coping mechanisms.

Moreover, the psychological impact of floaters can affect relationships. Individuals may find themselves withdrawing from social interactions due to embarrassment or discomfort with their visual condition. Friends and family may not fully understand the distress caused by floaters, leading to feelings of frustration and loneliness for the affected person.

Building a supportive network is essential in managing these emotional challenges, as open communication can foster understanding and provide reassurance to those struggling with the psychological ramifications of floaters.

Addressing the emotional and psychological aspects of living with floaters is just as important as tackling the physical symptoms. Engaging in mindfulness practices, seeking therapy, or joining support groups can offer valuable tools for individuals feeling overwhelmed by their condition. Additionally, educating oneself about floaters and exploring effective strategies for eye health can empower individuals to take control of their situation.

By acknowledging the emotional journey associated with floaters, individuals can begin to heal not just their vision but also their overall psychological well-being.

Mindfulness and Relaxation Techniques

Mindfulness and relaxation techniques play a significant role in promoting overall eye health, particularly for individuals concerned about floaters. These practices can help reduce stress and tension, which are known to exacerbate many eye-related issues.

By incorporating mindfulness and relaxation into daily routines, individuals can achieve a greater sense of calm and awareness, allowing for better management of their symptoms. Focusing on the present moment can also shift attention away from floaters, providing a mental reprieve that may contribute to a more positive outlook on eye health.

One effective mindfulness technique is deep breathing. This simple practice involves inhaling deeply through the nose, allowing the abdomen to expand, and then exhaling slowly through the mouth. Deep breathing helps activate the body's relaxation response, reducing the production of stress hormones that can negatively impact eye health.

Practicing this technique for just a few minutes each day can create a sense of tranquility, making it easier to cope with the anxiety that often accompanies floaters. It is beneficial to establish a routine that includes deep breathing, perhaps in the morning or before bedtime, to foster consistency.

Meditation is another powerful tool for enhancing mindfulness and relaxation. Engaging in regular meditation sessions can help individuals cultivate a deeper awareness of their thoughts and feelings.

This awareness can lead to a more accepting attitude toward floaters, reducing the fixation on them. Various forms of meditation, such as guided imagery or body scan techniques, can provide a structured approach to relaxation.

By focusing on different parts of the body during meditation, individuals can release tension and promote a sense of well-being, which may indirectly support eye health.

Yoga is also an excellent practice that combines mindfulness with physical movement. Specific yoga poses can improve blood circulation and reduce stress, contributing to overall eye health. Incorporating gentle stretches and poses that promote relaxation can be particularly beneficial for individuals dealing with floaters. Additionally, the emphasis on controlled breathing in yoga can further enhance relaxation and mindfulness. Engaging in a regular yoga practice, even for a short duration, can create lasting benefits for both the mind and body.

Lastly, it is essential to create a calming environment that supports mindfulness and relaxation efforts. Dimming the lights, reducing noise, and eliminating distractions can help foster a peaceful atmosphere conducive to these practices. Incorporating elements such as soothing music, essential oils, or nature sounds can enhance the relaxation experience.

By dedicating a specific space for mindfulness and relaxation, individuals can cultivate a sanctuary that promotes healing and well-being, ultimately supporting their journey in managing floaters and improving their overall eye health.

Building a Support Network

Building a support network is an essential step for those dealing with eye floaters. Connecting with others who share similar experiences can provide emotional support, practical advice, and valuable insights into coping mechanisms.

Whether through online communities, local support groups, or social media platforms, engaging with others can alleviate feelings of isolation and fear associated with floaters. Understanding that you are not alone in your journey can be profoundly reassuring and empowering.

Online forums and social media groups dedicated to eye health are excellent starting points for building a support network. These platforms allow individuals to share their stories, discuss treatment options, and exchange tips on managing floaters. Participating in discussions can help you gain diverse perspectives on coping strategies and the impact of floaters on daily life.

Additionally, these communities often feature members who have successfully navigated similar challenges and can offer encouragement and hope.

Local support groups can also play a crucial role in fostering connections among individuals dealing with floaters. Many cities have organizations focused on eye health that host meetings and events. These gatherings provide an opportunity to meet others face-to-face, share experiences, and learn from one another. Establishing relationships in person can enhance the emotional support you receive, allowing for deeper connections and a sense of community that online interactions may not fully provide.

Healthcare professionals can be a valuable part of your support network as well. Eye care specialists, therapists, and holistic practitioners can offer insights and advice on managing floaters. They can help create a comprehensive approach to your eye health, incorporating both traditional and alternative treatments. Building a relationship with your healthcare team encourages open communication, ensuring that you feel comfortable discussing your concerns and exploring various strategies for relief.

Finally, family and friends are integral members of your support network. Communicating openly about your experience with floaters can foster greater understanding and empathy among loved ones. They can provide emotional support, help you navigate challenging times, and even accompany you to appointments.

By sharing your journey with those close to you, you create a more supportive environment that can significantly enhance your overall well-being as you work towards healing and managing floaters effectively.

How To Heal Floaters

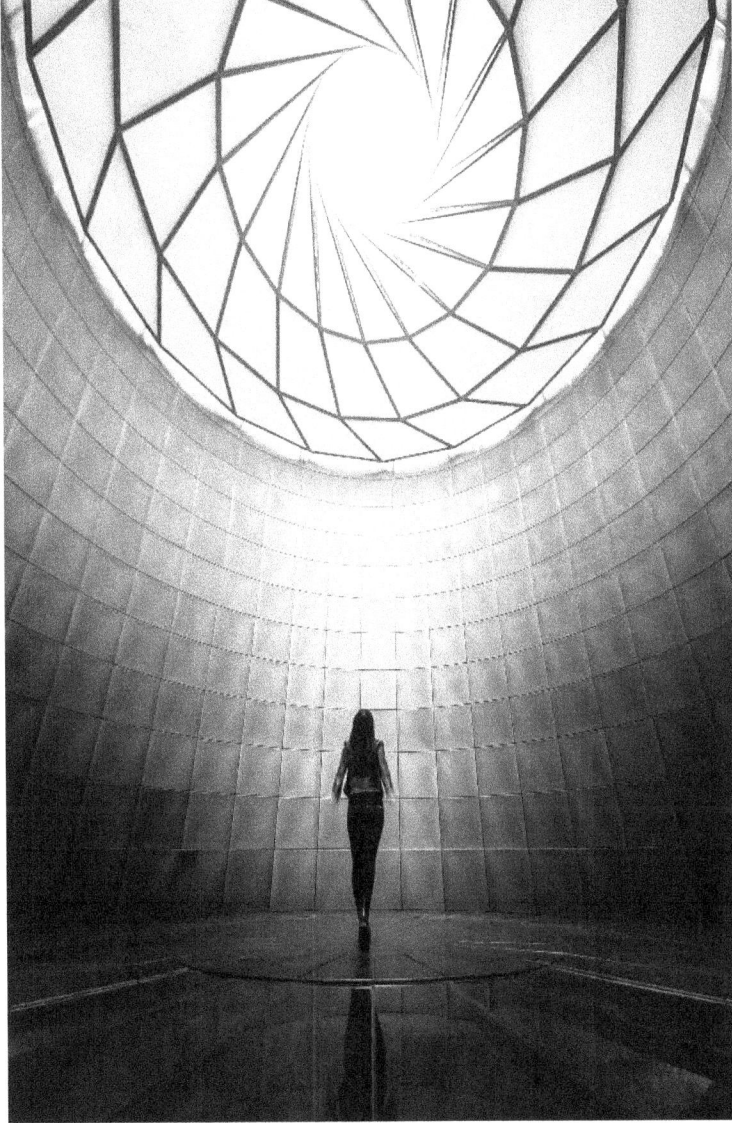

Chapter 10

Future Research and Innovations

Advances in Eye Care Technology

Recent advancements in eye care technology have significantly transformed the way we diagnose and manage various ocular conditions, including floaters. These advancements not only enhance our understanding of the eye's anatomy and physiology but also improve the efficacy of treatments available for floaters.

Technologies such as high-resolution imaging, optical coherence tomography (OCT), and advanced laser therapies are pivotal in providing deeper insights into the causes of floaters and tailoring personalized treatment plans for patients.

High-resolution imaging techniques have revolutionized the assessment of the vitreous gel in the eye. These imaging modalities allow eye care professionals to visualize the vitreous and any associated changes in detail, aiding in the identification of floaters' origins.

By employing these techniques, practitioners can differentiate between benign floaters and those that may indicate more serious conditions, such as retinal tears or detachments. This capability is crucial for early intervention and can significantly influence the outcome for patients experiencing floaters.

Optical coherence tomography (OCT) stands out as a particularly valuable tool in the management of floaters. This non-invasive imaging technology provides high-resolution, cross-sectional images of the retina and the vitreous. By using OCT, clinicians can assess the structural integrity of the vitreous and detect any abnormalities that could contribute to the formation of floaters.

Additionally, OCT can help monitor changes over time, allowing for more informed decisions regarding treatment options and the necessity for surgical intervention if the floaters are affecting the patient's quality of life.

In recent years, advanced laser therapies have emerged as viable treatment options for persistent floaters. These minimally invasive procedures utilize lasers to break apart the floaters, making them less noticeable and less intrusive to the patient's vision. Laser vitreolysis, for instance, has gained popularity for its ability to target and treat floaters without the need for invasive surgery. Patients who have undergone this procedure often report significant improvements in their visual comfort, thereby alleviating the distress caused by floaters.

As technology continues to evolve, the future of eye care holds promise for even more innovative solutions for managing floaters. Ongoing research into gene therapy, regenerative medicine, and advanced surgical techniques may lead to groundbreaking treatments that address the underlying causes of floaters rather than merely alleviating their symptoms.

For individuals concerned about floaters, staying informed about these advances is essential, as they may offer new hope and effective strategies for enhancing eye health and overall quality of life.

Potential Breakthroughs in Treatment

Recent advancements in medical research have opened new avenues for addressing eye floaters, a common yet often frustrating condition. Traditional treatments have primarily focused on management strategies rather than definitive solutions.

However, emerging technologies and innovative approaches are beginning to show promise in offering more effective treatment options. These breakthroughs not only aim to reduce the visibility of floaters but also address the underlying causes of their formation in the vitreous gel of the eye.

One of the most significant developments in treating floaters is the use of laser vitreolysis. This technique involves using a focused laser beam to break apart the floaters, effectively reducing their size and visibility. While this procedure has been available for some time, recent improvements in laser technology have enhanced its safety and efficacy. Clinical studies have indicated that patients experience substantial reductions in floater symptoms, with many reporting a marked improvement in their quality of life following the treatment.

Another area of exploration is the use of pharmacological interventions. Researchers are investigating various compounds that may help dissolve or alter the composition of the vitreous gel, potentially preventing floaters from forming or reducing their prevalence.

Early trials with these medications show encouraging results, although further research is required to assess their long-term effectiveness and safety. If successful, these treatments could provide a non-invasive option for individuals who prefer to avoid surgical interventions.

Gene therapy represents a groundbreaking frontier in the treatment of floaters. By targeting specific genetic markers associated with the development of floaters, scientists are exploring the possibility of modifying the biological processes that lead to their formation. While still in the experimental stages, the potential to alter the vitreous environment on a molecular level could revolutionize the way floaters are treated, offering a more permanent solution rather than temporary relief.

In addition to these medical advancements, lifestyle modifications and preventive measures are gaining recognition as vital components of floater management. Research continues to explore the impact of nutrition, hydration, and eye exercises on eye health. Integrating these strategies with emerging treatments could enhance overall effectiveness and lead to a more comprehensive approach to managing floaters.

As understanding of this condition evolves, the future appears promising for those seeking relief from floaters, with a combination of innovative treatments and holistic strategies paving the way for improved eye health.

Staying Informed on Eye Health Trends

Staying informed about eye health trends is crucial for individuals concerned about floaters. The field of eye health is continuously evolving due to advancements in research, technology, and treatment options.

By keeping up with the latest developments, individuals can make informed decisions regarding their eye care and explore new strategies for managing floaters. Engaging with credible sources of information, such as medical journals, reputable websites, and healthcare professionals, can provide valuable insights into the current understanding of floaters and potential remedies.

One significant trend in eye health is the growing emphasis on preventive care. Many eye specialists are advocating for regular eye examinations as a means to detect potential issues early, including floaters.

Understanding the risk factors associated with floaters, such as age, eye trauma, and certain medical conditions, enables individuals to take proactive steps to protect their vision. By staying informed about these factors, individuals can better communicate with their healthcare providers and develop personalized strategies to maintain their eye health.

Technological advancements are also reshaping the landscape of eye care. Innovations such as optical coherence tomography (OCT) allow for more precise imaging of the eye, helping professionals assess the condition of the vitreous humor and identify changes that may lead to floaters.

Additionally, new treatment options, including minimally invasive procedures, are being researched and implemented. Staying abreast of these advancements can empower individuals to discuss potential treatments with their eye care specialists and explore options that may best suit their needs.

Moreover, peer support and community engagement play a vital role in staying informed about eye health trends. Online forums, support groups, and social media platforms provide spaces for individuals to share their experiences, insights, and questions related to floaters.

Engaging with a community can help individuals feel less isolated in their concerns and provide access to shared knowledge about managing and potentially alleviating floaters. Such connections often lead to the discovery of helpful resources and support networks that can enhance one's journey toward better eye health.

Lastly, maintaining a holistic approach to eye health is increasingly being recognized as beneficial. This involves not only staying informed about floaters but also understanding the impact of lifestyle choices on overall eye health. Diet, exercise, and stress management have been linked to eye health outcomes.

Being aware of how these factors influence floaters can encourage individuals to adopt healthier habits. By integrating this knowledge into daily life and remaining vigilant about eye health trends, individuals concerned about floaters can take significant steps toward better vision and overall wellness.

Author Notes & Acknowledgments

First and foremost, I would like to express my deepest gratitude to the people who inspired and supported me throughout the journey of writing this book. This project would not have been possible without their unwavering belief in me and their invaluable contributions.

To my wife, thank you for your constant encouragement and understanding. Your love and support have been my anchor during the challenging times of researching and writing this book. Your belief in my ability to make a difference in people's lives has been my driving force.

I would also like to disclose that this book contains some renewed artificial intelligence-generated content. I really appreciate very recent technological innovation by outstanding scientists and of course our reader's understanding.

Lastly, I want to express my deepest gratitude to the readers of this book. I sincerely hope the strategies and methods outlined within these pages will provide you with the knowledge and tools needed to truly make your life much better. Your commitment to seeking any good solutions and willingness to explore multiple methods is commendable.

Author Bio

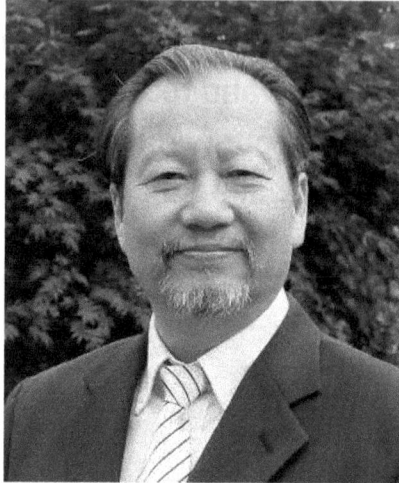

Johnson Wu earned his MD in 1982. With over 40 years of clinical experience, he has worked in hospitals in Zhejiang and Shanghai, China, as well as the Royal Marsden Hospital (part of Imperial College) in London, UK. Upon the recommendation of Sir Aaron Klug, the president of The Royal Society and a Nobel Prize winner in Chemistry, Dr. Wu was honorably awarded a British Royal Society Fellowship. He has published over 100 medical books in many countries and currently practices medicine in Canada.

www.ingramcontent.com/pod-product-compliance
Lightning Source LLC
Chambersburg PA
CBHW060250030426
42335CB00014B/1644